NAMASTE
Notebook

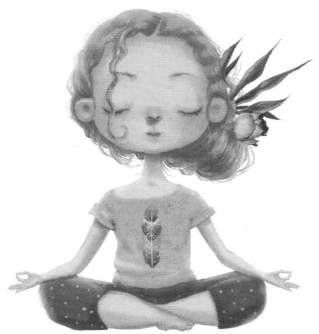

A Ruled Notebook With A Goal Planner And A Yoga Pose Chart

This Notebook Belongs To:

_____

E-mail:

Phone:

GOALS:

- [ ]
- [ ]
- [ ]
- [ ]
- [ ]
- [ ]
- [ ]
- [ ]
- [ ]
- [ ]

Accomplishments:

- ○
- ○
- ○
- ○
- ○
- ○
- ○
- ○
- ○
- ○

Habit Tracker	1	2	3	4	5	6	7	8	9

Appointments & Special Dates:

TREE

MOUNTAIN

HALF MOON

HANDS TO HEART

CHAIR

SEATED TWIST

STANDING SEPARATE LEG
HEAD TO KNEE POSE

WARRIOR I

WARRIOR II

EXTENDED SIDE ANGLE

CAMEL

HALFWAY LIFT

FORWARD FOLD

RAG DOLL

COW

CAT

CORP

SLEEPING HERO

CHILD

BOW

DOWNWARD-FACING DOG

COBRA

PLANK

LUNGE

TREE

MOUNTAIN

HALF MOON

HANDS TO HEART

CHAIR

SEATED TWIST

STANDING SEPARATE LEG
HEAD TO KNEE POSE

WARRIOR I

WARRIOR II

EXTENDED SIDE ANGLE

CAMEL

HALFWAY LIFT

FORWARD FOLD

RAG DOLL

COW

CAT

CORP

SLEEPING HERO

CHILD

BOW

DOWNWARD-FACING DOG

COBRA

PLANK

LUNGE

TREE

MOUNTAIN

HALF MOON

HANDS TO HEART

CHAIR

SEATED TWIST

STANDING SEPARATE LEG
HEAD TO KNEE POSE

WARRIOR I

EXTENDED SIDE ANGLE

CAMEL

HALFWAY LIFT

FORWARD FOLD

RAG DOLL

COW

CAT

CORP

SLEEPING HERO

CHILD

BOW

DOWNWARD-FACING DOG

COBRA

PLANK

LUNGE

TREE

MOUNTAIN

HALF MOON

HANDS TO HEART

CHAIR

SEATED TWIST

STANDING SEPARATE LEG
HEAD TO KNEE POSE

WARRIOR I

WARRIOR II

EXTENDED SIDE ANGLE

CAMEL

HALFWAY LIFT

FORWARD FOLD

RAG DOLL

COW

CAT

CORP

SLEEPING HERO

CHILD

BOW

DOWNWARD-FACING DOG

COBRA

PLANK

LUNGE

TREE

MOUNTAIN

HALF MOON

HANDS TO HEART

CHAIR

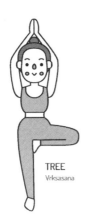

TREE
Vrksasana

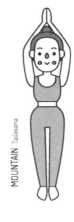

MOUNTAIN Tadasana

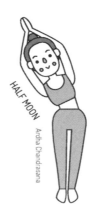

HALF MOON Ardha Chandrasana

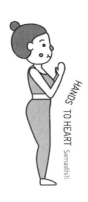

HANDS TO HEART Samasthiti

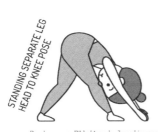

STANDING SEPARATE LEG
HEAD TO KNEE POSE

Dandayamana-Bibhaktapada-Janushirasana

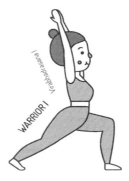

WARRIOR I Virabhadrasana I

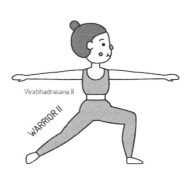

Virabhadrasana II

WARRIOR II

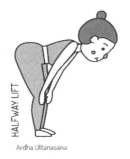

HALFWAY LIFT

Ardha Uttanasana

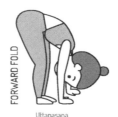

FORWARD FOLD

Uttanasana

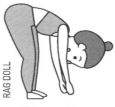

RAG DOLL

Uttanasana variation

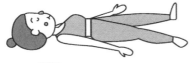

CORP Savasana

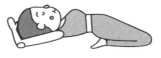

SLEEPING HERO Supta Virasana

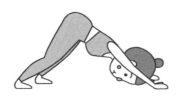

DOWNWARD-FACING DOG Adho Mukha Svanasana

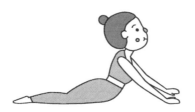

COBRA Bhujangasana

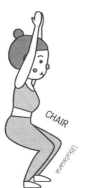

CHAIR
Utkatasana

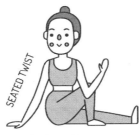

SEATED TWIST
Marichyasana III

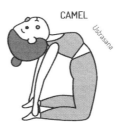

EXTENDED SIDE ANGLE
Utthita Parsvakonasana

CAMEL
Ustrasana

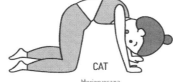

COW
Bitilasana

CAT
Marjaryasana

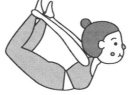

CHILD   Balasana

BOW   Dhanurasana

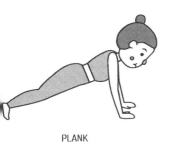

PLANK

LUNGE   Ashva Sanchalanasana

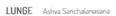

NAMASTE

BONUS!!!
Link to download free PDF version of
"Color Your Butterflies Away"

https://rwsquaredmedia.wordpress.com/free-coloring-book/

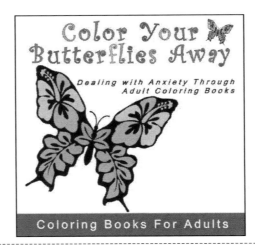

For inspirational prints and posters, visit:

https://InspirationalWares.com

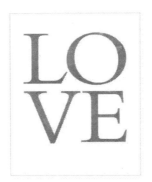
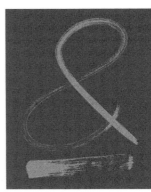
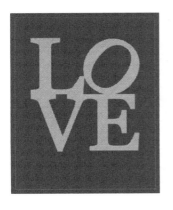
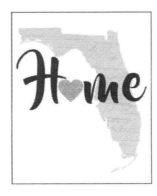
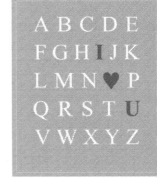

For more amazing journals and adult coloring books from RW Squared Media, visit:
Amazon.com
CreateSpace.com
RWSquaredMedia.Wordpress.com

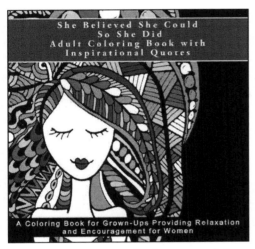

She Believed She Could
So She Did
Adult Coloring Book

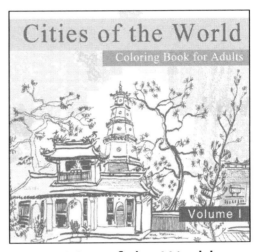

Cities of the World
Coloring Book for Adults

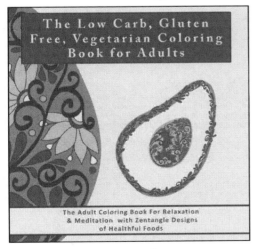

The Low Carb, Gluten Free,
Vegetarian Coloring Book for
Adults

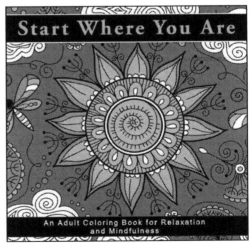

Start Where You Are
Adult Coloring Book

Made in the USA
Middletown, DE
31 October 2019

77696987R00062